HERBAL ANTIBIOTICS AND TREATMENT

Treatment for 69 common sickness and diseases

By

ANNANTRAM A. DIVINE

COPYRIGHT

TABLE OF CONTENTS

INSOMNIA (SLEEPLESSNESS)
RASHES ON PRIVATE PARTS
SWOLLEN LEG IN PREGNANT WOMAN)
BREAST CANCER
BODY ODOUR
PNEUMONIA
VIRGINAL DISCHARGE
FAST HEART BEAT
SWOLLEN LIVER
LOST VOICE
MENSTRUAL PROBLEM
POISON
TOOTH ACHE IN ADULT
NOSE BLEEDING
CURE FOR MALARIA FEVER
TYPHOID FEVER
CHEST PAIN
DIABETES
STOMACH ULCER
BED WETTING
RHEUMATISM AND ARTHRITIS
CHILDREN CONVULSION
TO REGAIN STRENGTH
WEAKNESS OF ERECTION OF PENIS
ASTHMA
MALARIA IN PREGNANT WOMEN

SEVERE HEADACHE
WORM IN STOMACH
EYE PROBLEM
RUNNING STOMACH
EAR DISEASE
PIMPLES
ABDOMINAL PAIN AFTER DELIVERY
SIGHT AND EYES RELATED PROBLEM
CURE OF FIBROID
TUBERCULOSIS
COUGH
INTERNAL PILE
EXTERNAL PILE
DIFFICULT BREATHING IN NEW BORN
BABY
MEASLES
VENEREAL DISEASE
SNAKE AND SCORPION BITE
SNAKE BIT AT BUSH
MEMORY IMPROVEMENT
STROKE
WOUNDS
HOW TO STOP VOMITING
YELLOW FEVER
HOW TO CURE HEAT IN THE WOMAN
STOMACH

INTRODUCTION

Welcome to the world of herbal medicine! This book is a comprehensive guide to the vast and fascinating world of medicinal herbs, their uses, and their benefits. Herbal medicine is an ancient practice that has been used for centuries to treat a wide range of ailments, from minor cuts and bruises to chronic illnesses.

In this book, you will discover the power of nature's healing plants and learn about their traditional and modern applications. You will also find information on how to identify, grow, harvest, and prepare herbs for medicinal use, as well as recipes for herbal remedies and tips for incorporating herbs into your daily routine.

Whether you are a seasoned herbalist or a newcomer to the world of natural healing, this book has something for everyone. So join us on this journey through the world of herbal medicine and unlock the incredible healing potential of nature's pharmacy.

PART ONE

HERBAL TREATMENTS

 The application of various plant parts is the basis of herbal medicine. parts of the plant that can be used medicinally.

The stem, fruits, seeds, flowers, and roots are all examples of these parts.

The chemical compounds that the plants naturally contain are what give them their medicinal properties.

These synthetic compounds are the supplements that make up for the lack of the synthetic compounds when they are brought into the body. Herbal medicine can be used for both prevention and treatment.

We eat a lot of vegetables, so herbs are basically vegetables. Food would indeed have become our medicine and medicine our food if we ate them with the intention of avoiding disease.

Natural medication is one of the most established types of medication on the planet. In fact, it has been extensively researched and documented in some nations.

Moving closer to home, various African nations have utilized a wide variety of herbs to treat a variety of ailments for a considerable amount of time.

In Nigeria, herbal medicine has a problem because it is not well documented. Specialists all around the nation have passed on not having recorded the information on Home grown medication for relatives.

As I observe a lot being produced by current practitioners, I have no doubt that this trend is about to change.

Home grown medication has been polished and utilized for the treatment of various afflictions for quite a long time.

Nature has favored mankind with an enormous number of various spices, Loaded down with gigantic measures of restorative properties that can be conveyed for the treatment and counteraction of various diseases.

Benefits of Herbal Medicine The rate at which herbal medicine is becoming more and more popular is alarming, to put it mildly. Additionally, it is vital to take note of that this prevalence of home grown medication as it is today, is upheld by substantial proof and declarations.

This only adds credence to what scientists like Dr. Batmangheldj had long asserted. He said the human body being Nature must be restored by Regular substances and not by inorganic compound medications.

Benefits of herbal medicine include:

1. Herbal products are affordable and cost-effective: Pharmaceutical products and modern medical practices are becoming so expensive that the average person cannot afford them.

Herbal medicine has emerged as a viable alternative to modern medicine due to the growing body of evidence demonstrating its increasing efficacy and significantly lower incidence of side effects.

2. Home grown items in type of enhancements, natural teas, separate medicinal oils, etc, are not difficult to obtain. They are accessible in wellbeing food shops, jumping up out of control and on the Web and drug store shops.

Additionally, because they are derived from plants, you do not require a prescription to purchase them. Likewise supplements don't need to be enlisted by the FDA in America and they don't need to go through preliminaries before use.

Nevertheless, as consumers, we must ensure that we purchase products from reputable retailers. Additionally, the items should be fabricated and bundled from legitimate organizations. Always ensure that you carefully read the labels on the supplements' bottles and packets.

3. The effectiveness of these herbs in treating a variety of illnesses has been established. Their efficacy has been demonstrated by numerous studies.

In fact, some herbs can be used to treat mild conditions like the common cold, while others can be used to treat more serious conditions like diabetes, cancer, and cardiovascular diseases.

4. Helping the insusceptible framework: Products made from herbs don't affect how the body works physiologically. They, on the other hand, encourage such procedures.

Particularly, the chemical components of herbal products boost the immune system. They make the system work better by working with every part of it. By providing sufficient antioxidants, for instance, they support the antioxidant immune system.

Some Native Medicinal Herbal plants

1. Moringa leaf
2. Lime leaf and fruit
3. Cymbopogon citratus (lemon grass)
4. Mango bark
5. Pawpaw leaf (papaya leaf)
6. Ocimum gratissimum (scent leaf)
7. Zingiber (ginder)
8. Allium sativum (garlic)

- **MORINGA LEAF**:

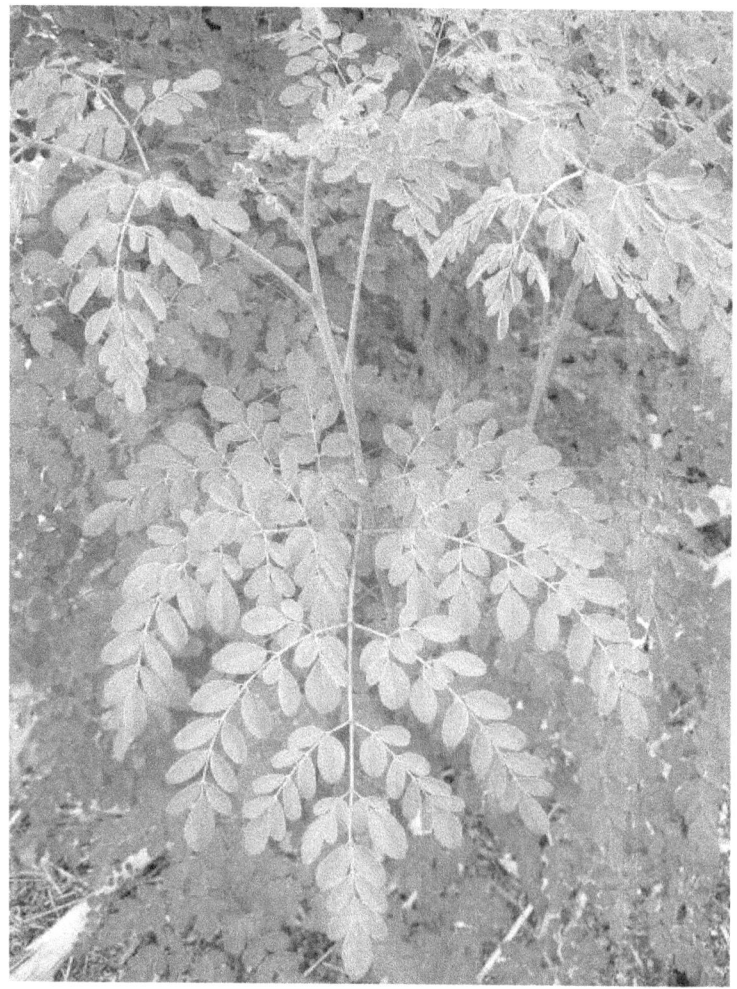

The plant Moringa is also known as the horseradish tree, the miracle tree, the drumstick tree, and the ben oil tree.

Due to its medicinal properties and health benefits, moringa has been used for centuries. Additionally, it has anti-inflammatory, anti-fungal, and antiviral properties.

Moringa contains numerous empowering mixtures, for example,

vitamin A, vitamin B1 (thiamine), vitamin B2 (riboflavin), vitamin B3 (niacin), vitamin B-6 (folate), vitamin C (ascorbic acid), calcium, potassium, iron, magnesium, phosphorus, and zinc.

Due to its medicinal properties and health benefits, moringa has been used for centuries. Additionally, it has anti-inflammatory, anti-fungal, and antiviral properties.

How does moringa work?
Moringa has healing properties and a wide range of beneficial compounds.

Moringa contains numerous beneficial compounds, including:

vitamin A, vitamin B1 (thiamine), vitamin B2 (riboflavin), vitamin B3 (niacin), vitamin B-6 (folate), vitamin C (ascorbic acid), calcium, potassium, iron, magnesium, phosphorus, and zinc.

What are the advantages?
Moringa is used for a variety of purposes, including health and beauty, disease prevention, and treatment. Moringa's benefits include:

1. Moringa seed oil is good for the skin and hair because it protects them from free radicals and keeps them clean and healthy. Moringa helps to protect skin cells from damage because it contains protein. Additionally, it has elements that hydrate and cleanse the body, both of which benefit the hair and skin.

It may be effective in treating wounds and infections of the skin.

2. Treatment of edema Edema is a painful condition in which fluid builds up in particular body tissues. Moringa's anti-inflammatory properties may be able to stop edema from developing.

3. Moringa appears to protect the liver from damage caused by antitubercular medications and can speed up the liver's repair process.

4. Treatment and prevention of cancer Moringa extracts have properties that may aid in the development of cancer. Additionally, it contains niazimicin, a substance that prevents cancer cells from growing.

5. Moringa extracts may be beneficial in the treatment of some stomach disorders, including gastritis, ulcerative colitis, and constipation. Moringa's antibacterial and antibiotic properties may assist in preventing the growth of various pathogens, and its high vitamin B content aids in digestion.

6. Moringa extracts may be used to treat infections caused by Salmonella, E. coli, and

Rhizopus due to their antibacterial, antifungal, and antimicrobial properties.

7. Healthier bones Moringa also has calcium and phosphorus in it, which help keep bones strong and healthy. Moringa extract may be used to treat arthritis and heal broken bones in addition to its anti-inflammatory properties.

8. Moringa is thought to be helpful in treating depression, anxiety, and fatigue as mood disorders.

9. Safeguarding the cardiovascular framework The strong cell reinforcements found in Moringa concentrate could assist with forestalling cardiovascular harm and has likewise been displayed to keep a solid heart.

10. Extract of moringa has been shown to aid in the healing of wounds and reduce the appearance of scars.

11. Moringa helps treat diabetes by lowering blood glucose levels and the levels of sugar and protein in the urine. This superior the

hemoglobin levels and generally protein content in those tried.

12. Moringa for asthma treatment may prevent bronchial constrictions and lessen the severity of some asthma attacks. It has also been demonstrated to improve overall breathing and lung function.

13. Safeguarding against kidney issues Individuals might be less inclined to foster stones in the kidneys, bladder or uterus assuming that they ingest moringa extricate. The high antioxidant content of moringa may help lower kidney toxicity levels.

14. Moringa contains compounds called isothiocyanate and niaziminin that help to prevent arteries from thickening, which can raise blood pressure.

15. Healthier eyesight Moringa's high antioxidant levels have the effect of improving eyesight. Moringa may prevent capillary membrane thickening, inhibit retinal

dysfunction, and stop the dilation of retinal vessels.

16. Moringa may help a person with sickle cell disease and anemia absorb more iron, thereby increasing their red blood cell count. The plant extract is thought to be very helpful in treating and preventing sickle cell anemia..

NOTE: Any native herbal treatment containing Moringa should not be taken by pregnant women or those hoping to conceive, it has antifertility properties.

- **LIME LEAF AND FRUIT**

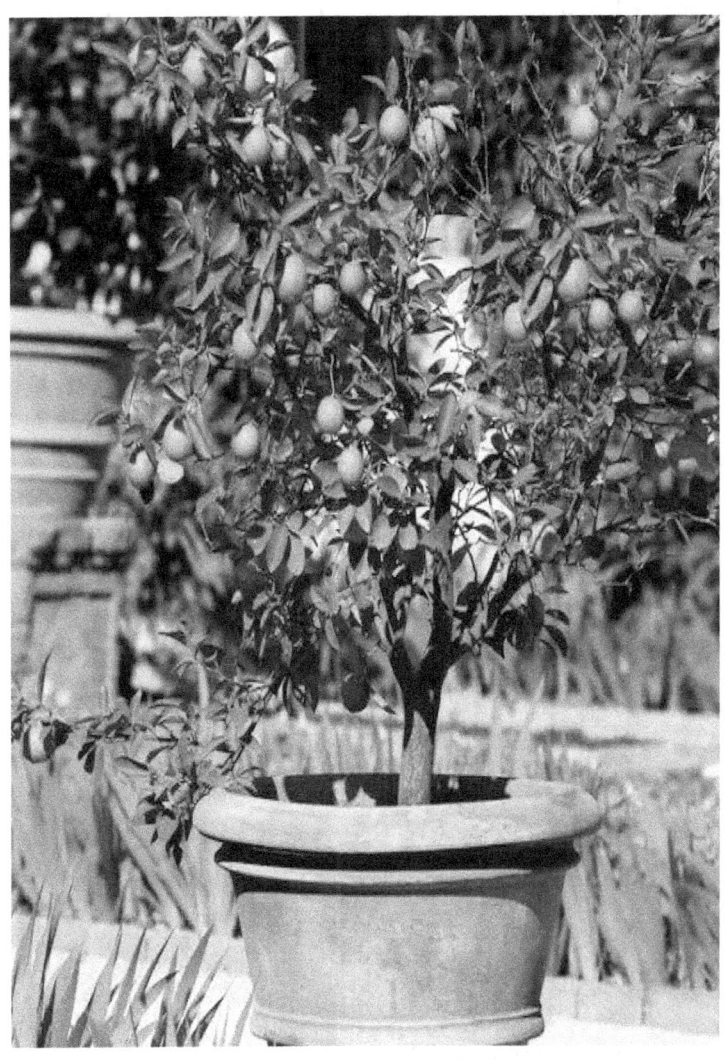

1. Limes are a type of citrus fruit, along with lemons, oranges, and grapefruits. They are small and round with a bright green skin.

2. Limes are rich in vitamin C, which is important for immune health, skin health, and wound healing.

3. Lime juice is acidic and has a tart, tangy flavor. It is commonly used in cooking, baking, and cocktails.

4. Limes are a good source of antioxidants, which help to protect the body from damage caused by free radicals.

5. Key limes, also known as Mexican limes, are smaller and more acidic than regular limes. They are often used to make Key lime pie.

6. Lime essential oil is sometimes used in aromatherapy to promote feelings of relaxation and reduce stress.

7. Limes are often used in traditional medicine to treat a variety of ailments, including coughs, colds, and digestive issues.

8. Limes are low in calories and high in fiber, making them a good choice for people trying to manage their weight or improve their digestive health.

9. The juice and zest of limes can be used to add flavor to a variety of dishes, including salads, marinades, and desserts.

10. Limes are grown in many different parts of the world, including Mexico, India, and the United States. They are harvested year-round and are most commonly available in the summer months.

Limes (fruit) are a nutritious fruit that can provide a number of health benefits. Here are some of the main health benefits of consuming limes:

- Rich in vitamin C: Limes are an excellent source of vitamin C, which is a powerful antioxidant that helps protect the body against damage from free radicals. Vitamin C is also important for immune function, skin health, and wound healing.

- Boosts immune system: The high vitamin C content in limes can help to boost the immune system and reduce the risk of infections, such as colds and flu.

- Supports digestion: Limes are a good source of fiber, which is important for digestive health. The citric acid in limes can also help to stimulate the production of digestive juices, which can aid in the digestion of food.

- Promotes hydration: Limes are rich in water, which makes them a great choice for staying hydrated. Adequate hydration is important for many aspects of health, including skin health, kidney function, and overall energy levels.

- May reduce inflammation: The antioxidants found in limes, such as vitamin C and flavonoids, have anti-inflammatory properties. This means that consuming limes may help to reduce inflammation in the body, which is associated with a range of chronic diseases.

- May lower risk of chronic disease: The antioxidants found in limes may help to reduce the risk of chronic diseases, such as heart disease, diabetes, and cancer.

- Supports skin health: The vitamin C content in limes can help to promote collagen production, which is important for maintaining healthy skin. Limes may also have antibacterial properties that can help to reduce the risk of skin infections.

Lime leaves are the leaves of the lime tree (Citrus aurantifolia), and they are commonly used in Southeast Asian cuisine for their aromatic flavor. Here are some of the potential health benefits of lime leaves:

- May have anti-inflammatory properties: Lime leaves contain compounds that have anti-inflammatory properties, which means they may help to reduce inflammation in the body. Chronic inflammation is linked to a range of health issues, including heart disease, diabetes, and cancer.

- May have antibacterial properties: Some studies have suggested that lime leaves may have antibacterial properties, which means they could help to fight off harmful bacteria in the body. This could potentially reduce the risk of infections.

- May have antioxidant properties: Lime leaves contain antioxidants, which can help to protect the body against damage from free radicals. Free radicals are molecules that can damage cells and contribute to the development of chronic diseases.

- May aid in digestion: Lime leaves have been traditionally used in Southeast Asian medicine to aid digestion. They may help to stimulate the production of digestive juices and promote healthy digestion.

- May improve heart health: Some studies have suggested that compounds found in lime leaves may help to reduce cholesterol levels and improve blood pressure, which could lower the risk of heart disease.

- **CYMBOPOGON CITRATUS (LEMON GRASS)**

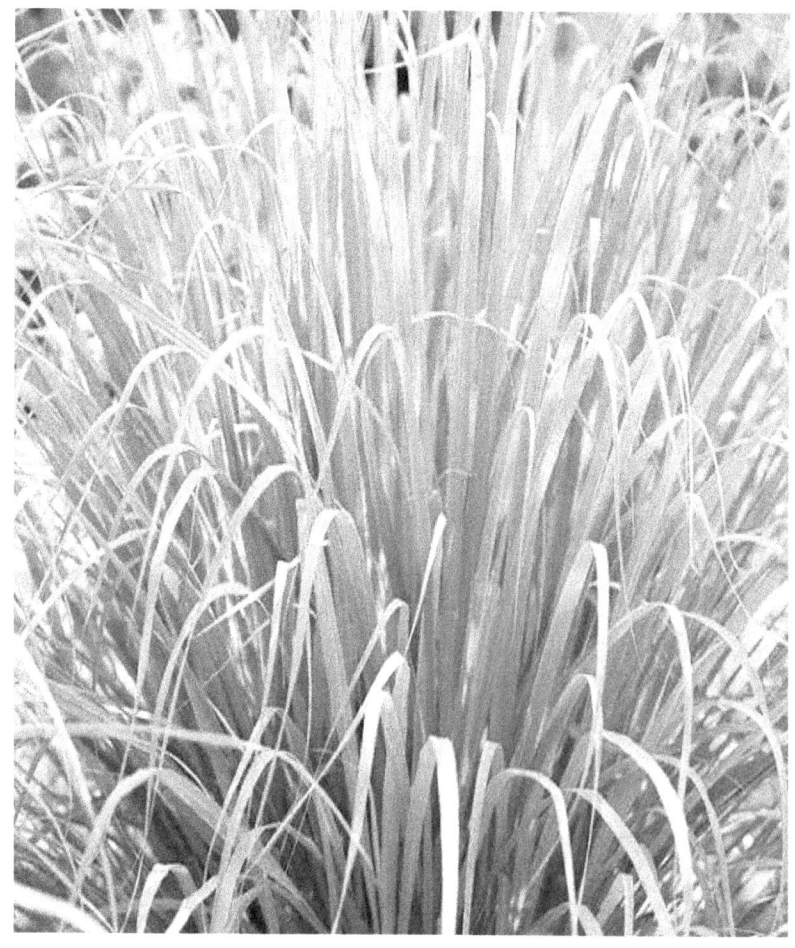

Lemongrass (Cymbopogon citratus) is a tropical herb that is commonly used in cooking and traditional medicine. Here are some of the potential health benefits of lemongrass:

1. May reduce inflammation: Lemongrass contains compounds that have anti-inflammatory properties, which means it may help to reduce inflammation in the body. Chronic inflammation is linked to a range of health issues, including heart disease, diabetes, and cancer.

2. May have antibacterial properties: Some studies have suggested that lemongrass may have antibacterial properties, which means it could help to fight off harmful bacteria in the body. This could potentially reduce the risk of infections.

3. May aid in digestion: Lemongrass has been traditionally used in traditional medicine to aid digestion. It may help to

stimulate the production of digestive juices and promote healthy digestion.

4. May have antioxidant properties: Lemongrass contains antioxidants, which can help to protect the body against damage from free radicals. Free radicals are molecules that can damage cells and contribute to the development of chronic diseases.

5. May have anti-anxiety properties: Some studies have suggested that lemongrass may have anti-anxiety properties, which means it could help to reduce feelings of anxiety and promote relaxation.

6. May improve skin health: Lemongrass contains compounds that have anti-inflammatory and antimicrobial properties, which means it may help to improve skin health and reduce the risk of skin infections.

7. May reduce fever: Lemongrass has been traditionally used in some cultures to

reduce fever. It may have a cooling effect on the body and help to reduce body temperature.

It's worth noting that more research is needed to fully understand the potential health benefits of lemongrass

• MANGO BARK

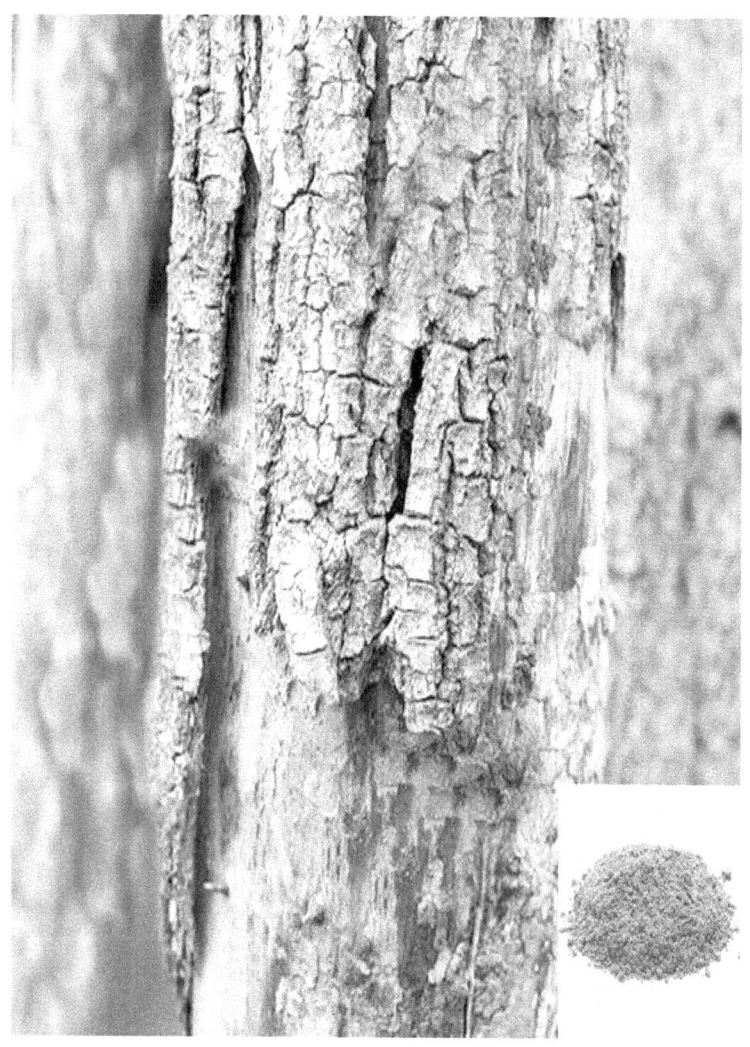

The bark of the mango tree (Mangifera indica) has been traditionally used in some cultures for medicinal purposes. However, it is important to note that the use of mango bark for medicinal purposes is not widely studied, and more research is needed to fully understand its potential health benefits and risks.

Some traditional uses of mango bark include:

- Treating diarrhea: The bark of the mango tree has been traditionally used in some cultures to treat diarrhea. It is believed to have astringent properties, which means it may help to reduce inflammation and tighten the tissues in the intestines.

- Treating fever: In some cultures, mango bark has been used to reduce fever. It is believed to have a cooling effect on the body and may help to reduce body temperature.

- Treating respiratory problems: Mango bark has been traditionally used in some cultures to treat respiratory problems, such as coughs and bronchitis. It is believed to have expectorant properties, which means it may help to loosen mucus and make it easier to cough up.

- Treating pain: Mango bark has been traditionally used to treat pain, such as toothaches and headaches. It is believed to have analgesic properties, which means it may help to reduce pain.

- **PAWPAW LEAF (PAPAYA LEAF)**

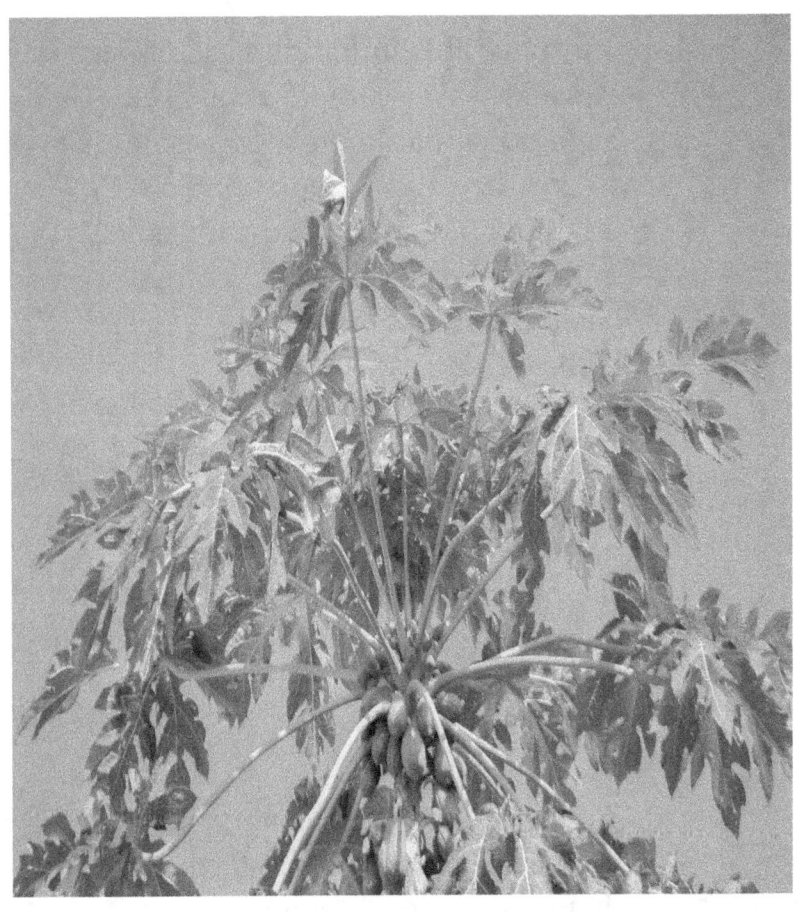

Pawpaw leaves (Carica papaya) have been traditionally used in some cultures for their potential health benefits. Here are some of the potential health benefits of pawpaw leaves:

1. May have anti-inflammatory properties: Pawpaw leaves contain compounds that have anti-inflammatory properties, which means they may help to reduce inflammation in the body. Chronic inflammation is linked to a range of health issues, including heart disease, diabetes, and cancer.

2. May have antioxidant properties: Pawpaw leaves contain antioxidants, which can help to protect the body against damage from free radicals. Free radicals are molecules that can damage cells and contribute to the development of chronic diseases.

3. May have antibacterial and antiviral properties: Some studies have suggested that pawpaw leaves may have antibacterial and antiviral properties,

which means they could help to fight off harmful bacteria and viruses in the body. This could potentially reduce the risk of infections.

4. May help with digestion: Pawpaw leaves have been traditionally used to aid digestion. They may help to stimulate the production of digestive enzymes and promote healthy digestion.

5. May have anticancer properties: Some studies have suggested that pawpaw leaves may have anticancer properties, which means they could help to prevent or slow the growth of cancer cells.

6. May have antimalarial properties: Some studies have suggested that pawpaw leaves may have antimalarial properties, which means they could help to prevent or treat malaria.

- **OCIMUM GRATISSIMUM (SCENT LEAF)**

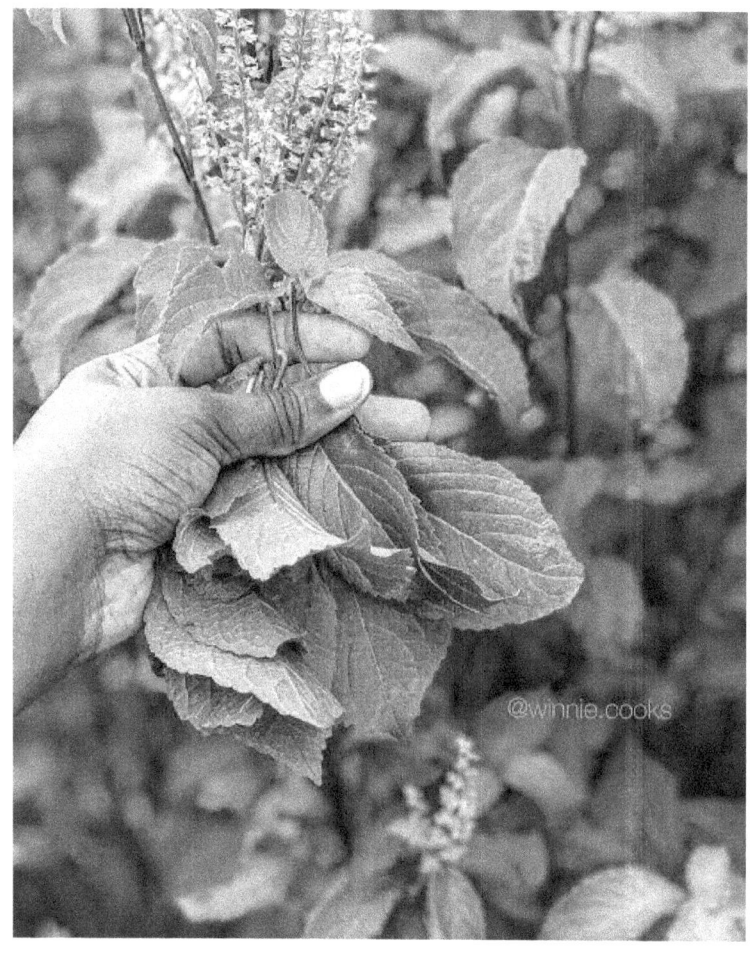

Scent leaf, also known as Ocimum gratissimum, is a tropical plant that is commonly used in cooking and traditional medicine in many parts of the world. Here are some of the potential health benefits of scent leaf:

1. May reduce inflammation: Scent leaf contains compounds that have anti-inflammatory properties, which means it may help to reduce inflammation in the body. Chronic inflammation is linked to a range of health issues, including heart disease, diabetes, and cancer.

2. May have antimicrobial properties: Scent leaf has been traditionally used to fight off harmful bacteria and fungi. Some studies have suggested that it may have antimicrobial properties that could help to prevent infections.

3. May help with digestion: Scent leaf has been traditionally used to aid digestion. It may help to stimulate the production of

digestive juices and promote healthy digestion.

4. May help with respiratory issues: Scent leaf has been traditionally used to treat respiratory problems, such as coughs and colds. It may have expectorant properties, which means it may help to loosen mucus and make it easier to cough up.

5. May have antioxidant properties: Scent leaf contains antioxidants, which can help to protect the body against damage from free radicals. Free radicals are molecules that can damage cells and contribute to the development of chronic diseases.

6. May help with pain relief: Scent leaf has been traditionally used to treat pain, such as headaches and toothaches. It may have analgesic properties, which means it may help to reduce pain.

● ZINGIBER (GINDER)

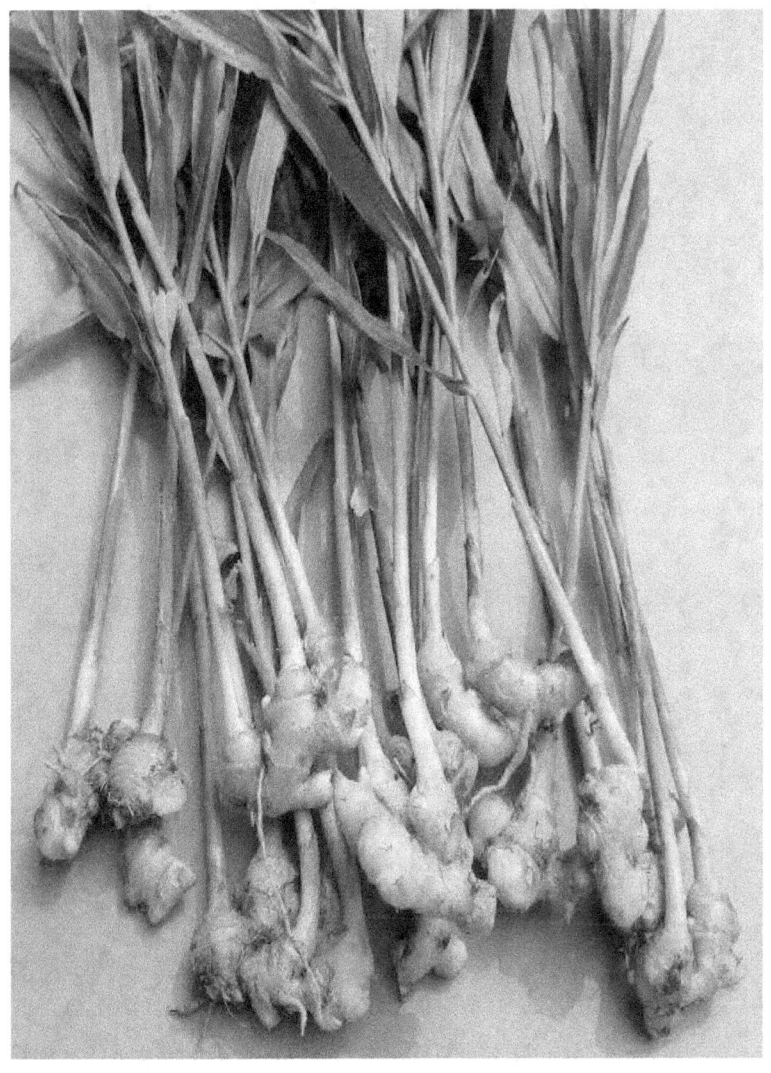

Ginger (Zingiber officinale) is a spice and medicinal plant that has been used for thousands of years in many cultures for its potential health benefits. Here are some of the potential health benefits of ginger:

1. May help with nausea and vomiting: Ginger has been shown to be effective in reducing nausea and vomiting, particularly in pregnant women and people undergoing chemotherapy or surgery.

2. May reduce inflammation: Ginger contains compounds that have anti-inflammatory properties, which means it may help to reduce inflammation in the body. Chronic inflammation is linked to a range of health issues, including heart disease, diabetes, and cancer.

3. May help with digestion: Ginger has been traditionally used to aid digestion. It may

help to stimulate the production of digestive juices and promote healthy digestion.

4. May help with pain relief: Ginger has been shown to have analgesic properties, which means it may help to reduce pain, particularly in people with osteoarthritis.

5. May help with blood sugar control: Some studies have suggested that ginger may help to lower blood sugar levels, which could be beneficial for people with diabetes.

6. May have antioxidant properties: Ginger contains antioxidants, which can help to protect the body against damage from free radicals. Free radicals are molecules that can damage cells and contribute to the development of chronic diseases.

- **ALLIUM SATIVUM (GARLIC)**

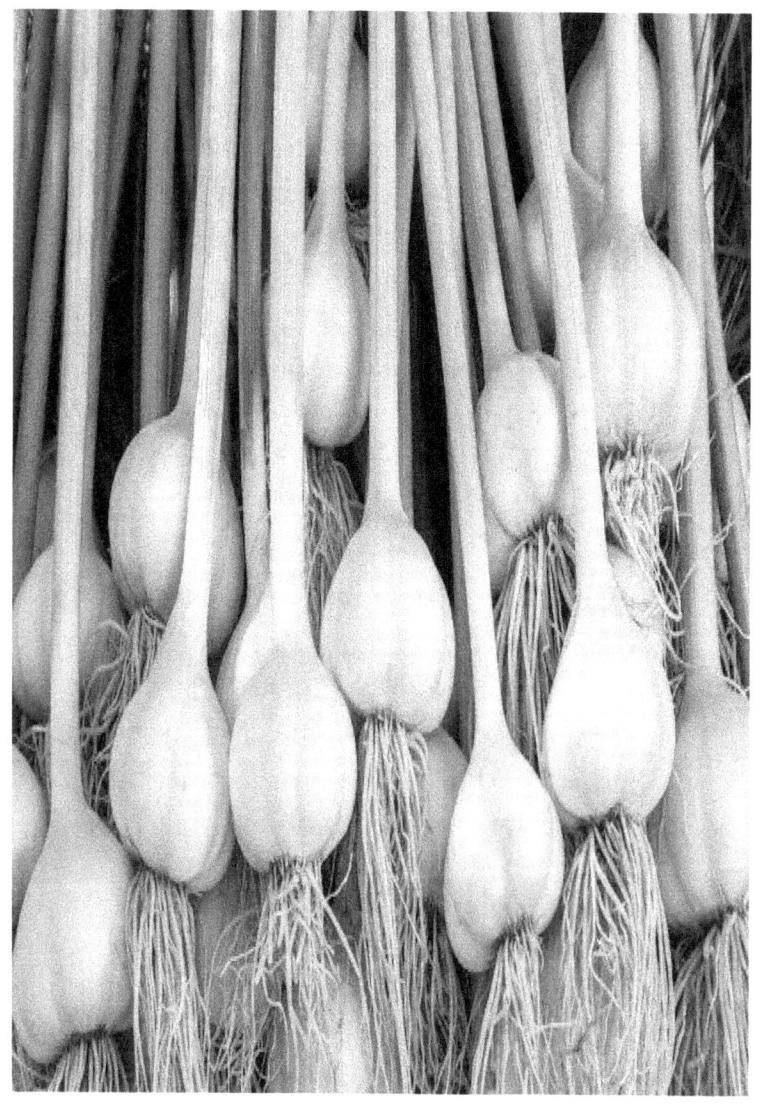

Garlic has been traditionally used for its medicinal properties for centuries, and modern research has confirmed many of its health benefits. Here are some of the potential health benefits of garlic:

1. May lower blood pressure: Garlic may help reduce blood pressure by relaxing the blood vessels and improving blood flow. This can potentially reduce the risk of heart disease and stroke.

2. May reduce cholesterol levels: Garlic may help reduce levels of LDL cholesterol, also known as "bad" cholesterol, which can accumulate in the arteries and increase the risk of heart disease.

3. May have anti-inflammatory effects: Garlic contains compounds that may help reduce inflammation in the body, which can contribute to chronic diseases like arthritis, cancer, and heart disease.

4. May boost the immune system: Garlic has antimicrobial properties and may

help strengthen the immune system, potentially reducing the risk of infections.

5. May have anticancer properties: Some studies suggest that garlic may have anticancer properties, potentially reducing the risk of certain types of cancer, such as stomach, colon, and breast cancer.

OUR TRADITIONAL BREWED MEDICINE
99% EFFECTIVE

Here in Africa Africa before the arrival of modern medicine, we already had the herbal or rather traditional method of curing and treating most sickness and diseases, but for the sake of gilboa book, I will be telling us a method to treat and prevent

Malaria
Fever
Indigestion
Reduce inflammation
Boost immune system
Lower blood pressure
Antibacterial

As you observed above I gave a list of only 8 herbs just because of this purpose, and all have similar health benefits.

Below is the combination of herbs that help treat and prevent the above mentioned sickness or diseases, and also boost your immune system against them.

1. Moringa leaf: pluck an arm length of a branch of the tree.
2. Lime leaf and fruit: also an arm length branch for the leaf and slice open four lime in equal halves.
3. Pawpaw or papaya: add two or one branch depending on how big it is.. Just the leaf, not the stem holding the leaf.
4. Mango Bark: A handful of mango Bark, Adult hands
5. Lemon grass: five stems or should I say branches or strands..anyone you understand.
6. Scent leaf: Also an adult hand compressed full.
7. Garlic: Just one, slice it
8. Ginger: just one slice it

Preparation

Add all the above measurements in the appropriate quantity into a pot, and add water to cover the herbal mix. Then let it boil for 30 mins without opening the pot (so add enough water)

(Note: you can add or reduce measurement depending on your required quantity).

Usage

There are two ways of using this mixture
- External
- Internal

1. **EXERNAL**:

   This can be done by sitting on a low stool with the pot (unopened) then covered air tight with a big bedspread or duvet so the steam from the heated herbal mixture does not escape, Then you open the pot and stir with a spoon to allow the vapor of the herbal pot heat up your body stay in the heat for 5 mins to 10 mins so that the mixture can soak into your body.

2. **INTERNAL**:

   Drink One tea cup full of the herbal mixture at a warm temperature.

This can help cure all the illnesses mentioned above and can also help to prevent them too and it's 99% effective.

Health is wealth, treat yourself before you get worse..

PART TWO

HERBAL EASY TREATMENT TO 69 COMMON ILLNESS OR DISEASES

1. Miscarriage

If woman is having constant miscarriages or she is seeing her menstruate while pregnant, she should drink two (2) spoon of pure noney for morning and evening throughout her pregnancy.

2. BLEEDING AFTER DELIVERY

This had lead to the death of many women. Although there are injection that can stop such bleeding but when the environment or area has no such treatment or delivering take place in wrong hour, people may be confused, living the woman to bleed to death.
HERBAL REMEDY: Collect rotten Plantain Pseudo and press the water inside a cup and give it to the bleeding patient to drink, immediately the bleeding will stop.

3. RING WORM

Mix pure honey with lemon orange juice then rub on the affected part.

4. CHOLERA (STOOLING & VOMITING)

HERBAL REMEDY: Collect one short of gin and one tea spoon of sugar and salt. To be taken.
Or
Take some gari in plate and pour gin inside let the gin cover the garri then drink the garri the vomiting and stooling will stop. This will be done only when someone is in condition, but not for children.
N.B: If you drink gin and eat dry gari in your mouth it will dry your mouth and it could lead to seizing of breath which could be dangerous So soak inside the gin and drink it wet not separately

5. EASY LABOUR (QUICK DELIVERY)

Squeeze plenty of Gorchorus Olitorus (Ewedu -leaves.in Yoruba) in water and filter. To be taken during abour.

6. EPILEPSY

The whole day fresh urine should be take until one Is relieved of the problem but not for a woman having Menstruation

7. NIGHT BLINDNESS

This is due to lack of Vitamin A. Food such as vegetables, Fruits, milk and liver should be eaten by the person...

8. INSOMNIA (SLEEPLESSNESS)

Honey mix with Aloe Vera juice to be taken in the night, it will help relax the body and take you to sleep.

9. RASHES ON PRIVATE PARTS

Squeeze bitter leafand scent leaf together. To be rubbed well on the effected parts, you can also drink the solution ½ glass three times daily.

10. SWOLLEN LEG IN PREGNANT WOMAND

Get much quantity of corn silk boil in water and Sweeten with honey.
DOSSAGE: Take one glass regularly until situation improves

11. BREAST CANCER

Get three big yam head and grind. One cup of honey and one Aloe Vera juice: Rub it on the breast, Aloe Vera juice should be put in water to be taken at least one time a week.

12. BODY ODOUR

Grind the flower of African lavender mix with lime and soap. Bath with the mixture regularly.

13. PNEUMONIA

Mix 12 Lime and juice of 3 grapes ferment all with grinded garlic onions. Take a shot of it and a table spoon of honey.

14. VIRGINAL DISCHARGE

Wash the virginal with a maximum of warm water, native soap and lime orange juice.
N. B: the affected patient should take half glass of palm wine in the morning and evenig for a week.

15. FAST HEART BEAT

Collect 7 Avocado Pear seed and mango leaf, then boil. Take a cup 3 times daily.

16. SWOLLEN LIVER

Get about 12 unripe mangos in a pot and add water. Boil for some time and allow to cool, then filter and mix with a cup of honey. Take two shot twice daily.

17. LOST VOICE

Boil water and collect one cup from it. Add 2 teaspoonful of honey into of the hot water; open your mouth and inhale the heat into your mouth do this 4 times daily.

18.   MENSTRUAL PROBLEM

SYMPTOMS: irregular flow of blood from the uterus, characterize by several pain in the abdomen, body irritation and dullness.
HERBAL REMEDY
1.If appears as in abdominal pain, collect bitter leaf and squeeze with little water, add small potash to be taken during the pain, Morning and evening
2. If appear's as irregular and disorder, get a tea infusion of mistletoes leaf and drink 1 cup 3 times a day it will correct irregularities and disorder.

19. POISON

If any one has been poisoned by any substance
either by food or by drinking e.g. Kerosine.
Instant poison, the following should be apply

HERBAL REMEDY:Grind Charcoal and mix it
with cooled water, force the person being
poisoned to drink it. The Charcoal will absorb
and collect the poison substance into the navel
and be passed out as excretes.

20. TOOTH ACHE IN ADULT

i.Get a half cup of warm water and drop an
Alum in it. The warm water will malt the Alum,
then turn it inside your mouth and direct the
warm water mix with Alum Into the affected
tooth. Cover the mouth for a few seconds. Pour
out the water and repeat it again for two or
three times. Do this for 3 days Tooth problem
will be
solved

ii.peel the back of coconut and put it inside a
small pot, add small salt with a little water, boil

the solution for some time and drop. After cooling a little, pour it inside the mouth and direct the hot solution to the affected tooth to heat the gum for some time. Do this 3 times a week.

21. NOSE BLEEDING

Squeeze basil or scent leaves and allow the drop into the nose. The bleeding will stop.

22. CURE FOR MALARIA FEVER

Get Guava leaves, Paw-paw leaves and Dogoyaro leaves. peel back of mango tree; Cut some lemongrass and add lime orange (7) cut all into pieces and add 4 liters of water in a pot, boil it for about 40 mins. Remember to warm daily DOSAGE: Half a cup three times daily. After food.

23. TYPHOID FEVER

Grind one bulb of onions, a bunch of garlic onions and soak with a little clean water, look for basil (Curie leaves) and lemongrass, squeeze together and add the water to the onion and garlic you first soak. Take half glass in the morning and in the evening for 10 days. Do this on a daily basis, the fever will disappear.

N. B.: Typhoid Fever always takes blood. The patient should wash vegetable leaves (pumpkin leaf) and warm it to be drunk regularly.

24. CHEST PAIN

Get 7 Avocado pear seed pieces and dry in sun grind and keep for treatment. DOSAGE: 2 tablespoons of pap (Akamu) every morning. Only one week you will notice a change and for one month the pain is gone

25. DIABETES

Collect bitter leaf and scent leaf and squeeze with a little water, filter and grind Garlic onion in it and warm it. To be taken in the morning and in the evening for one month DIABETES will disappear, your urine will turn salty and excess urination will stop

N.B. Do this on a daily basis.

26. STOMACH ULCER

This is an open sore in the stomach
CAUSES: starvation, hot food, too much pepper and salt etc.

HERBAL REMEDY: Get about 12 of unripe plantain peel off the coat, slice and pound it, soak with 4 liters gallon of water, cover it for 3 days, then drink the water regularly.
N.B: Immediately you start drinking the water, you should avoid eating heavy food such as: Eba, Santana also known as Akpu, pounded yam and beans the patient should be taking light food such as, Rich, Tea, Bread, Pap e.t.c

27. BED WETTING

The child that is up to 12-15 years of age is not supposed to urinate on bed.
HERBAL REMEDY: collect bitter leaf and scent leaf squeeze with little water filter it and drink. Do this in the morning and evening for one month. The bladder that is too open will be

adjusted to accurate position and BED WETTING problem will be solved

28. RHEUMATISM AND ARTHRITIS

This is the weakness and inflammation of joints. It is caused by some micro-organism which destroys some tissue thereby extending the pain to the bone marrow.
HERBAL REMEDY: collect 7 Avocado seed (English pear) pieces and dry in the sun. After dryness grind to powder and turn into an empty bottle fill the bottle with pure honey
DOSAGE: 2 spoons in the morning and in the evening.
N. B: Boa (Snake) oil should rub well on the joint but not around the private part.

29. CHILDREN CONVULSION

Every good mother should know these, as we all know convulsion is the worst enemy of children. You can help your neighbor with it, they will come and thank you later.

HERBAL REMEDY: Grind the cooking onions, Garlic onion and Ginger grind together mix with palm kernel oil (native oil).

Apply all over the body. Especially the Eyes, Mouth and Anus, convulsion will disappear.

30. TO REGAIN STRENGTH

Get 7 up or Sprite mineral mix with one teaspoon of salt and a tin of Peak milk and drink. Energy will come immediately.

31. WEAKNESS OF ERECTION OF PENIS

CAUSE:
1) Pile
2) Meeting woman under menstruation
3) Masturbation

HERBAL REMEDY: First treat yourself of pile. Get 6 big bulbs of onions. Cook half done, grind and squeeze and collect the juice, filter and mix with an equal amount of pure honey stir and warm.

DOSAGE: 2 spoons in the morning and in the evening for a week.

32. ASTHMA

This is an inability to breathe normally, which is caused by too much Cool weather. The weather has been too cool which results in inflammation of the respiratory organs thus making breathing very difficult.

HERBAL REMEDY: collect the white fluid of snail and add equal amount of pure honey, Mix and pour into a bottle.

DOSAGE: 2 tablespoon 3 times daily.

Or

Mix half a glass of pure honey and onion juice together to be taken every day for one month.

33. MALARIA IN PREGNANT WOMEN

This is characterized by dullness and stretching of the body. The stretching of the body is not good for a pregnant woman, as it reduces the development of the pregnancy.

HERBAL REMEDY: Get some JUTE (EWEDU) stem and boiled with Water to be taken ½ glass at night.

34. SEVERE HEADACHE

Deep your legs into warm water for 3 minutes and after that you deep it again into cold water for 1 minute.

35. WORM IN STOMACH

Squeeze some Neem leaf (Dogoyaro leave) add 10 limes orange
DOSAGE: 1 spoon in the morning and evening for a week.

36. EYE PROBLEM

It is lack of Vitamin A
Use one bottle of pure honey and ½ Bottle of palm oil. Mix together to be taken a spoon a day.

37. RUNNING STOMACH

Mix a pure honey with orange juice DOSAGE: 2 spoonful 3 times daily.

38. EAR DISEASE

Ear discharge, Mucus or pimples or itching
i. hot water add little salt and honey inside and stir it, let one or two drop into the ear in the morning and evening when you are about going to bed. Do this for about one week.
ii. Get soldier ants atleast twenty Put it in a small bottle and add strong gin (local gin). Leave it for three days for the odour of the solider ant to mix with the gin properly. Insert the cotton wool into the small bottle and put two drop into the ear in the morning and evening for a week.

39. PIMPLES

CAUSE: Heat dirtiness and some oil in the face.
HERBAL REMEDY: Make sure you sponch your face with soap to remove dirty which might

have accumulate in the face as a result of oil in the face. Use lemon juice to wash your face every morning and apply the juice of Aloe vera every night on your face. The following morning make sure you wash it with sponch and sap before two week your face, will be so smooth as a baby face or skin.

40. ABDOMINAL PAIN AFTER DELIVERY

She has to take 2 spoon of honey 3 times daily for three months.
Then put honey in hot water and press the abdomen it.

41. SIGHT AND EYES RELATED PROBLEM

If the eye is itching you or the eye is looking red, it is as a result of worm in the eye.
HERBAL REMEDY: Wash your eye with your early morning urine or mix honey with onions and let two drop into the eye for three days, you can also squeeze tomatoes leaf or scent leaf

and let a drop into the eye. The worm that is itching or biting you, will withdraw to its normal position.

42. CURE OF FIBROID

Use white Kernel nut (unripe kernel). DOSAGE: Chew 25 nut each day for at least one month.

43. TUBERCULOSIS

Tuberculosis is a serious infective disease which associated with disorder of the lungs.
SYMPTOMS:
1. Difficult in breathing
2. Pain in the lungs
3. Deep throat cough.
HERBAL REMEDY: Grind 12 pieces of Bitter Kola, Ginger and Garlic onion mix the ingredient with a bottle of pure honey.
 ADULT 2 table spoon 3 times daily for a month.
N.B: Chew one bulb of Garlic onion before going to bed eat much fruits.

44. COUGH

Grind 12 pieces of Bitter Kola mix with a bottle of pure honey.
DOSAGE: Two (2) table spoon 3 times daily for a week.
or
Get Bitter Kola and burn, then grind it to collect the ashes, put in an empty bottle then add palm kernel oil into it and lick for a week

45. INTERNAL PILE

Squeeze bitter leaves, Scent leave and paw-paw leaves with water and add some lime then drink regularly.

46. EXTERNAL PILE

This is cause by eating unripe fruit.
HERBAL REMEDY: Get Indian herm generally know as Moroco. Dry the leaf and the seed and grind to powder, mix with native soap (black soap) add small hot water. Apply it gently to the anus. Before a week it will draw inside. After

that wash bitter leaf and give the water to the person to drink.

ii. Get warm water in a basin and add salt. The patient should sit on it for some seconds. Do this in morning and evening for a week. Definitely th pile problem will be solved.

47. DIFFICULT BREATHING IN NEW BORN BABY

During delivery, water can enter the baby's mouth which may lead to difficult breathing of the baby.

HERBAL REMEDY: Get lemon orange and collect the juice and give it to the new born baby to drink.

DOSAGE: One baby spoon in the morning, afternoon and evening for two days. The haby will vomit the water before breathing will be normal.

48. MEASLES

Apply natural undiluted honey on the body for the whole day

49. VENEREAL DISEASE

These can be transmitted either sexually or through public toilet e.g. Syphilis and Gonorrhea

HERBAL REMEDY: Tobacco leaf or two spoon of granulated one, pure into a big bottle and add 20 tetracycline (Red & Yellow Capsule) mix all with gin, cover and leave for 2 days to ferment. After 2 days take 3 shot glass in the morning and in the evening for 3 days, you will urinate the Gonorrhea out of your system.

N.B: Stomach Ulcer patient, pregnant mothers and nursing mothers should not drink the mixture

50. SNAKE AND SCORPION BITE

Get at least 7 bitter Cola grind and pour into a bottle, fill half of the bottle with palm Kernel Oil and five tablespoon full of an undiluted honey, mix all with one tin of milk and drink all the mixture you will vomit the poison

51. SNAKE BIT AT BUSH

If some one is at the bush or distant place from town or village, he can not get access to the above bitter Cola, Palm Kernel Oil and Honey as directed above, there is still some thing you can do to neutralize the poison. The person will get home safely pull out the centre leaf of a small palm tree and chew in a case where there is no palm tree, look for cassava and uproot, peel and eat to neutralize the poison of the snake.

N.B: You uproot cassava and eat, it will definitely neutralize the poison but do not drink water instantly, it is not good. it causes foam starches in the stomach and it could be dangervus to health.

52. MEMORY IMPROVEMENT

The kind of food a child eat when he was a baby contributes to the development of the brain. This is because the baby. needs a lot of Vitamin to build the brain for mental alertness, one of the substance that contains the Vitamin

is pure natural honey. Honey contains a lot that can help to Develop the brain properly.
DOSAGE: 2 in the morning and evening before the baby will be able to set properly. No doubt the child will grow up with a retentive memory.

53. STROKE

Collect 7 Avocado Pear seed, slice & dry it and grind together with mustered seed. Put it into a container & cover it. Take two tea spoon and mix with pap 3 times Daily for one month.

54. WOUNDS

To stop a bleeding wound get plantain or banana leave squeeze and apply the fluid on it. It will stop the bleeding. To dress a wound get lime and honey mix and apply it on the surface of the wound

55. HOW TO STOP VOMITING

Squeeze some quantity of scent leaves in water, filter and drink it at regular interval until symptom stop.

56. YELLOW FEVER

Get big unripe Paw-paw, peel off the body and remove the seed, slice the unripe Paw-paw and add cooled water.
DOSAGE: 1 table spoon 3 times daily.

57. HOW TO CURE HEAT IN THE WOMAN STOMACH

The heat can lead to infertility so treat yourself fast.
HERBAL REMEDY: 1 spoon of lime orange a day for one (1) month will clear the heat in the stomach.

58. EXCESS FLOW OF MENSTRUATION

Excess flowing of blood from the uterus during menstruation is very detrimental to the health. If a woman notice this, she should go to chemist store and buy vitamin K and drink it

59. DYSENTERY

CAUSES:

1)Dirty environment

2) Over-ripe fruit

3) Dirty water

4) Unripe fruit etc.

HERBAL REMEDY: take a glass of your urine every morning no matter how strong the dysentery is, it will stop. Urine is one of the extraordinary normal healing elements in the world.

60. DIARRHEA

Get cutting wool leaf (Gossypium arboreum) and wash with water and filter. Add 5 Tetracycline (red and yellow capsule) in a small bottle, while 10 if in a big bottle and shake property.

DOSAGE: one spoon in the morning and evening it will stop by two days.

61. HYPERTENSION (B.P)

Too much blood in the rain forcing the heart to over warm itself. Characterized by a very hard and fast heart beat to dizziness.

CAUSES: tension, too much thinking, obesity and smoking.

HERBAL REMEDY: Mistletoes leaves (parasites) it commonly found on an orange tree and Rubber tree e.t.c. It grows on top of any tree and any tree it grows on top, it kills the tree.

Do not try to leave under the sun because it reduces the nutrient but dry in cool, shaded dry place. Dry and grind for tea, DOSAGE: 2 spoons in a half cup warm water in the morning and evening.

N.B: Reduce your thinking.

ii. Grind one bulb of garlic onion and soak in a gin for a week to ferment for one week add coconut water and one bottle of pure honey take a shot of glass daily

62. MALARIA AND YELLOW FEVER]

This is active, if someone is being attacked by malaria or yellow fever, get a leaf known as Awhorhe oristse, Cut and squeeze enough lime orange in it. Add some salt, boil for some time then remove the leaf and drink the water. Do this for 3 days.

63. SEX WITHOUT PREGNANCY:

Due to ignorance, some girls have destroy their life with drugs abuse while some take acidic substances e.g. Lime orange mix with Potash and salt. The reason is that they do not want unnecessary pregnancy while some even go straight to abortion which is equal to murderer and against the sacrilege of marriage and to God Almiglity. After damaging their womb may will lay their problem on some one else. This drug abuse and Abortion can lead to tube blockage and low sperm count.

To help you, I was able to come out with a typic: "Sex Without Pregnancy"

SIGN OF OVULATION: the white discharge of eggs is a sure sign of Ovulation therefore, after such white discharge, the woman should give herself one week before having sex, if she doesn't want to get pregnant. Most women start Ovulating two weeks after the first day they see their menstruation. In such case the woman should put two weeks ahead immediately when she starts seeing her menstruation, it will fall on the ovulation period. What I am saying is that any day she starts seeing her menstruation should add 14 days. One week on the 14th is what we call a danger cave or peak period. Thpse are the days she will get pregnant if she has sex.

What I am saying in essence is that she should be adding 14 days to any first day she starts seeing her menstruation. If she sees it on the 10th she will add $10 + 14 = 24$. Then one week from the 24 to (24, 25, 27, 28, 29, & 30) is are dangerous days or peak period. If she starts seeing it on the 5th, she will add $5 + 14 = 19$ from on the 19 to 25 is a danger or peak period. The principal rule is whenever you notice sign of Ovulation, i.e. White discharge of eggs. Is clear evidence that Ovulation is approaching. Therefore, within the week after discharge are days the woman will get pregnant.

N.B: Some women see such signs of Ovulation 4 times a year. Such woman will find it difficult to get pregnant if she don't know this sign. So the woman should be watchful and wait for this signs. After this white discharge, she should has sex with her husband within that week

64. SICKLE-CELL (SICKLER)

Some parents had lost their child because of money to take care of them as a sickler. Your sickler child may be very well in the morning but in the afternoon or evening may be a different story. This is not the fault of the child, but the blood group the child got from the parent. Apart from spending money on a sickler, there is a way you can always make the child great. HERBAL REMEDY: get half part of an orange with a York of an egg, mix all together with one spoon of honey. Let the child do this on a daily basis. He or she will always be great.

65. MY GENERAL ADVICE

Some of the food we eat is very detrimental to health.

Eating fruit such as Paw-paw and mangos, the person should not drink any kind of minerals. It is very poisonous, it can leads to death or serious typhoid fever because the fruit has some acidic substance, when react with gas of the mineral, it will affect the heart. Another fruit that react negatively, is that of pepper fruit and any bear (Alcohol). It can affect your life. A person that eats Corn should not drink gin (Alcohol) as it is very harmful to one's life. Eating Wall-nut, the person should not drink a tablet immediately which could lead to death. A person that soaks garri and eat should not lick mangos instantly, it could Cause problems for the person.

66. CURE OF FIBROID & SEIZING OF MENSTRUATION

Grind mustard seed, mixed with olive oil 3 times daily for 28 days

Seizing of Menstruation:
Aloe vera leaf, slice into 10 litres container
Mixed with water to ferment for three days. And
take three times daily for one month.

67. CATARRH & COUGH

When someone's nostril is blocked, and unable
to breathe normally or if - the person has a dry
cough, he or she should put one TOMTOM in
his mouth while sleeping and when the
Tom-Tom melts off should quickly replace it with
another one before the day's break. Do this for
two days, you will easily cough out the catarrh
and that of your nostril will melt out.

68. EASY FLOW MENSTRUATION

If the menstruation is nor flowing well or it's
stopped, the woman should not wait for too
long because delay can lead to permanent
seizure of the menstruation.
HERBAL REMEDY: one spoon of Aloe-vera
juice into the glass of water, every morning for
seven day, when expecting the menstruation
but if the menstruation has seized she should

increase the dosage to two spoon of Aloe-vera juice into a glass of water

N.B: if the patient tries it for the first month and there is no good result she should repeat it.

69. APPENDICES AND HERNIA

1 bottle of gin, with 7 Alligator pepper and dry seed of pepper and tobacco leaf and 5 red and yellow capsules take it for 3 days.